I0711509

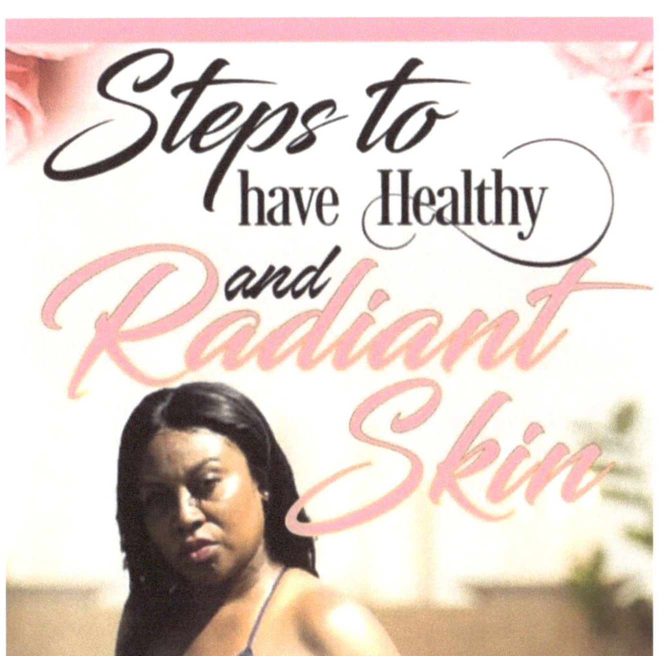
Steps to
have Healthy
and
Radiant
Skin

Steps to have Healthy and Radiant Skin

By LaWanda Keyes

www.theblessedessentials.com

2020

CONTENTS

LaWanda Keyes

Introduction

Isn't it time you pampered and babied your skin? I mean, why wouldn't you? It is the one organ that sells you out and speaks your confidence or the absence of it. This thing needs attention, and it needs it now.

Put everything aside, dearie.

This book gives you a rundown on how to serve the needs of your skin in five shorter-than-short chapters. It then shows you why each move is crucial, what to do, and what not to do.

Consider it a splendid thing that you are here. Every flip, slide or scroll will bring you in on the basics of healthy skincare.

Now dearie, shall we?

1. Sunning

The sun is a splendid star. It's a no brainer than the sun's rays bear the gift of Vitamin D.

Forget pharmaceutical drugs such as calcitriol, which supposedly have active vitamin D. I'm talking about nature's gold, side effects aside. Your body takes in the sun via your skin and makes the vitamin. Cool, right?

Why

- The fat-soluble vitamin prevents your skin from wrinkling. Therefore, you enjoy the smoothness and overall attractiveness and beauty.
- It promotes the repair and regeneration of skin cells.

- It is an anti-ageing element. We could say that it keeps you at sweet sixteen all your life.
- It has an immense microbial effect – it keeps your skin's immunity levels high. Organisms that find themselves in the wrong place under your skin get blown down to smithereens.

Dos

ℓ Expose your skin to at most half-an-hour of sunlight, preferably during mid-morning hours. Do this at least five times a week.

ℓ Use sunscreen if you have sensitive skin. No matter your skin tone, use the product if you're sunbathing at a high-index time (you know, the scorching sun).

Don'ts

ℓ Avoid spending too much sunbathing time if you're lighter (melanin-deficient). If you do, you may get a sunburn. Also, set limitations on sunlight exposure to your skin if it is sensitive. Worse comes to worst when they say that UV rays can cause cancer.

Ⓛ Avoid looking at the sun with your eyes. You wouldn't want eye damage, would you?

2. Feeding

They say we are what we eat, and what we take in shapes how we look. This mini-chapter will rush you through the foods and snacks you need to have flawless skin. And yes, you guessed it right – it is all organic.

Why

- Some foods have fatty acids, which form the basis of healthy skin cells.
- Other low-sugar snacks prevent glycation, a reaction that eventually gets your skin wrinkled.
- Others are antioxidants which help your inside to be toxin-free. In their expedition

around your body, they help maintain the suppleness of your skin.

- Many edibles improve your skin's toughness, making it more resistant to the effects of UV rays. Therefore, it becomes less susceptible to cancer.
- Other eatables have vitamins that up the production of your skin's oil.

Dos

- Eat more of the following affordable foods:

  - Kidney beans *for acne-free skin*
  - Avocados *for upping the vitamin levels in your dermis*
  - Oranges *to prevent skin-ageing*
  - Olive oil *for antioxidants – these mitigate the effect of free radicals*
  - Fatty fish such as salmon *for thickness*

- Snack on the following sugariness:

  - Organic dark chocolate *for firmness*

Don'ts

L Strictly avoid anything that may trigger an allergic reaction. It may have a lasting effect on your skin. For example, if you're lactose-intolerant, milk will disturb the stillness in the dermis and affect the surface's smoothness.

L If you can have it uncooked, then take it. It's richer that way.

3. Moisturizing

Dry skin doesn't feel flawless, or does it? Many people try to wrap their head around the dryness of their skin, but they often fail to get a way through. Here, I will open you up to the how-to of skin moisturizing. The read should make you feel impeccable. Trust me, you will.

Why

- Supple skin gives you a sense of confidence. That final look in the mirror before you step out then seeing your skin glowing charges you up.
- Moisturized skin helps to avoid the pain that comes with skin breakages. Have you ever had cracked lips which got extremely painful? Well, there's the point I am trying to make. Anyway, get some lip balm next time, dearie.

Dos

Know your type of skin. How oily or dry your skin naturally is determines its kind.

Pick a moisturizer. In the market, they are like the sand of the desert. Use the following to make your pick:

- How sensitive it is to your skin type

⚜ Whether it is oil-based, water-based, petroleum-based or medicinal, and if the component works for your skin type

⫿ Combine the moisturizer with a body wash (with jojoba, olive or coconut oil). It will help maintain and retain the skin's suppleness.

Don'ts

⫿ Avoid using moisturizing products before studying every ingredient used. You need to know all its nitty-gritty details.

⫿ Stop using other people's oils or ointments. You may confuse your skin, and I am sure that is the last thing you want.

4. Sleeping

It is sleep time, and now we want to shut our eyes and go to slumberland. Dermatologists have lauded sleep as a supplement for having healthier skin, and a healthier life. Coming out of an insomniac night makes one feel less energetic. That feeling trickles down to all our organs, including our skins. It is now time to see how sleep and skin correlate.

Why

+ Night-time is the skin's time to do some self-repair. At night, your body produces chemicals (from the food you had eaten earlier). The substances help to do away with dead skin cells and generate new ones.

- Blood flow is more active at night than during the day. The blood reaching your skin, full of oxygen, helps it to breathe anew.
- Proper sleeping helps you to avoid stress, which would otherwise produce a stress-induced hormone called cortisol. The hormone causes inflammation on your skin, thereby causing acne.

Dos

Ⅼ Master your day-night cycle. Know when your body tells you to sleep, and do it then for at least 7 hours.

Ⅼ If you're on your phone, use the night-light setting to lull your eyes to sleep. Spending too much time on your phone takes the zizz time away.

Ⅼ If you do not get sleep, book a full-body massage for yourself. It does not necessarily substitute your sleep, but it helps your body replenish and up its energy levels.

Have you ever heard about BEAUTY sleep? Take that as well!

Don'ts

◖ Avoid staying up too late. Let sleep time be just that - sleep time.

◖ Never see sleep as an item of inconvenience. You don't want it – you need it!

5. Treating

We will wrap up this skin business at a point of zenith – a point where we pamper our skins to death, or life, whichever it is. Your skin is as important as anything else, and it needs to feel cherished. Here, you and I will explore some skin treats. Dearie, time to love that skin!

Why

+ Skin treatment induces a feel-good feeling all over your body. Whatever the method, it always feels like you are in a state of nirvana.
+ The methods are as therapeutic to your skin as taking in the sun, eating well, moisturizing and sleeping tightly.

Dos

L Microdermabrasion is the removal of the skin's outermost surface. It helps to take care of age spots and acne.

L Facial misting. This method maintains the suppleness of your skin, especially during hot weather. You don't need to feel frazzled when you can stay cool using hydrating mist.

L Sauna sessions. Steam is potentially harmful, but it splendidly babies your skin. The sweat produced during the wet bath is a detoxifier. It flushes toxic bits and pieces that may be hiding under the skin's surface.

L Laser technology methods are resurfacing and rejuvenation. They help to remove damaged skin, initiating skin cell regeneration. Also, the technologies provide non-surgical ways of taking care of wrinkles.

Don'ts

L Avoid trying methods that you have not studied well to save yourself money and time.

L Avoid believing everything you see, read etc. Do your research and consult a dermatologist.

Conclusion

Well, that was it. After some eight pages, you can consider yourself a master of the art of skincare. *Flawless, Fleckless & Faultless: Your Skin is in Fine Fettle* has brought you to the attention of little and big things that should change the way you treat your skin.

Dearie, your skin is your baby, and it needs you all the time. I may be sounding corny, but that is how it is. If we saw the skin as an infant who needs constant, round-the-clock care, we would be looking, feeling and being different. We need to learn to love ourselves.

Now, I tell you to go and love your skin with a love that is more than love itself.

Toodles!

LaWanda Keyes